W0116083

CONTRADICTA *Aphorisms*

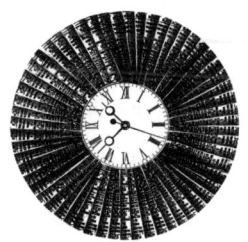

CONTRADICtA
aphorisms

by Nick Piombino

Illustrations by Toni Simon

GREEN INTEGER
KØBENHAVN & LOS ANGELES
2010

GREEN INTEGER BOOKS
Edited by Per Bregne
København / Los Angeles

Distributed in the United States by Consortium Book
Sales and Distribution / Perseus
www.cbsd.com (800-283-3572)
Distributed in England and throughout Europe by
Turnaround Publisher Services
Unit 3, Olympia Trading Estate
Coburg Road, Wood Green, London N22 6TZ
44 (0)20 88293009

(323) 857-1115 / http://www.greeninteger.com
Green Integer
6022 Wilshire Boulevard, Suite 202C
Los Angeles, California 90036 USA

First Green Integer Edition 2010
Copyright ©2010 by Nick Piombino
Art copyright ©2010 by Toni Simon
Back cover copy ©2010 by Green Integer
All rights reserved

Some of these aphorisms were previously published in *Boog City,
Eoagh, E-X-C-H-A-N-G-E-V-A-L-U-E-S, Green Integer Review,
Jacket, Or,* and *The Tiny.* The author wishes to thank the editors:
David Kirschenbaum, Tim Peterson, Tom Beckett, Douglas Messerli,
John Tranter and Elaine Equi, Paul Vangelisti, and Gina Myers and
Gabriella Torres

Design: Per Bregne
Typography: Rebecca Chamlee
Cover photographs: Photographs of Nick Piombino and Toni Simon

LIBRARY OF CONGRESS CATALOGING IN PUBLICATION DATA
Nick Piombino [1942]
Toni Simon (art)
Contradicta: Aphorisms
ISBN: 978-1-933382-48-7
p. cm – Green Integer 159
I. Title II. Series

Green Integer books are published for Douglas Messerli

Contradiction is not a sign of falsity, nor the lack of contradiction a sign of truth.

—BLAISE PASCAL

The philosopher thinks from eternity into the moment; the poet from the moment into eternity.

—KARL KRAUS
Dicta and Contradicta (1909)

It's the hidden things—like enigmas in dreams—that most often remind us that choices abound.

✷

Start at the beginning—then work back.

It's molting season: shed the old regrets and fly.

✳

Don't be too nicey to those who are icy.

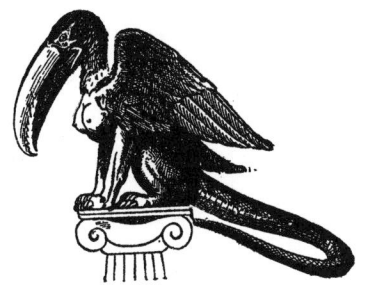

To be an artist is to be forever hungry for things you have never tasted, to relentlessly search for things you have never seen and can't understand, to repeatedly and warmly welcome back the most confused, lonely and unfair part of yourself, and the world. All for the singular joy of having something you can only experience by releasing it.

✳

Unforgettable music awakens abandoned hopes and forgotten dreams.

Little time to think about what you don't like or don't have when so much time is needed to think about what you can't understand.

✸

I fell asleep on a merry-go-round with a pocketful of tickets and woke up on a roller coaster with a handful of stubs.

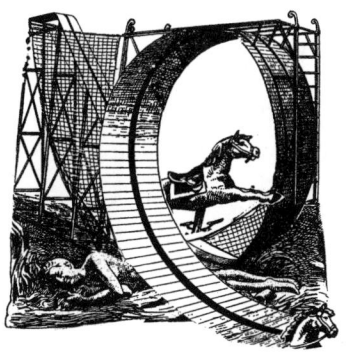

Understanding embodies the Midas touch. It mints the coin of knowledge out of the debris of loss.

✳

The precise force that at the proper time unbolts a portal at the wrong moment reveals a trap.

Courage is the stone, disappointment the river.

✳

Happiness is not the lack of sadnes; it is what sadness learns to wear in order to shine

Happiness is divulged with few words, misery demands a mouthful.

✳

In today's house I am the host, but I am a guest in the dwelling of yesterday.

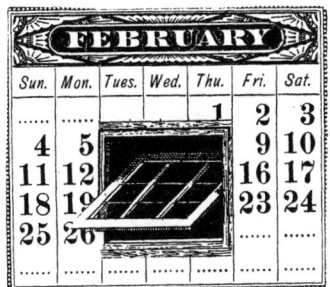

Contemptuous attitudes towards the rewards of old age—devoted spouse and friends, reputation, security, wisdom—spring easily from the mouths of the young, and, in fact, sound better coming from them.

✳

Despair over time passing is a quickening plunge that only insight can throttle.

Pleasing everyone pleases no one.

✳

Remember the future, forget the past.

Aphorisms remind us there is more to be understood in a world that suggests mostly there is more to be owned.

*

Everything can be known in an instant. That's all there ever was.

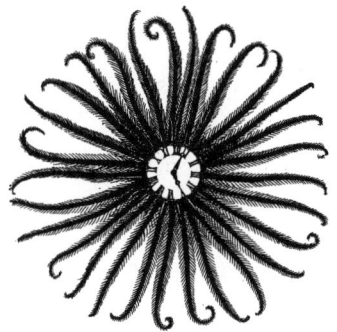

Measure detracts from pleasure.

＊

Until noticed, even the loveliest things feel plain.

Fools have the wit to agree on one thing: pay no attention to the wise.

＊

Among the greatest sources of happiness is to possess the means within to resist unhappiness.

One truth will produce a thousand lies, one kindness a thousand hurts, one success a thousand uncertainties.

*

Of all the potions, balms and drugs there is no more powerful elixir than a smile.

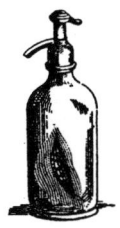

How many nascent ideas, skewered like game, lay dead at your feet?

※

Time wasted is time tasted.

Cruelty conquers briefly what kindness alone can keep.

❋

There is no escape: breathe deep.

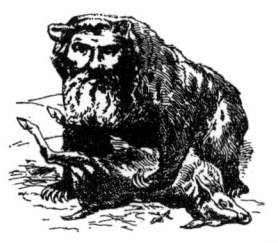

Acceptance of uncertainty won't banish every qualm but unreasonable demands for certitude will make doubt a steady companion.

＊

Not all information is beneficial. Cultivating a taste for not knowing some things may make for a better day.

First I embraced my doubts like they were my closest friends and they betrayed me. Then I learned to send them away quickly, with few words, like a known enemy, and they deceived me. Now I greet them warily and entertain them for awhile hoping to persuade them to tell me why they came. Until I extract their secrets—even if I banish and forget them —they will haunt me to the end of my days.

＊

You can't be sure until it's done but then how you did it is already a fading memory.

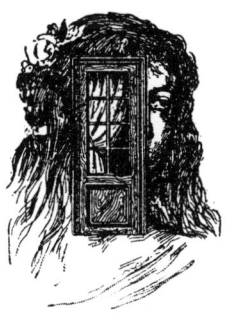

Waiting and thinking are enemies because when you are waiting you can think of nothing except what you are waiting for.

※

Suspense is fascinating—when it concerns what is happening to someone else.

The hoofbeats of uncertainty beat loudly on the road of destiny.

✳

The ship of fate favors a diligent captain with a good map and a strong stomach.

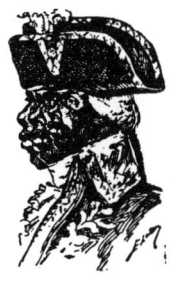

Thought is a delicate thing—nearly anything can interrupt or disturb it—particularly—as with most things—if you take too much at one time.

✳

Come to your own conclusions—or never see anything come to one.

People who have the least to say will try to silence others either by shouting them down or insulting them.

＊

Safer to kick a beehive than to malign a proud philosopher.

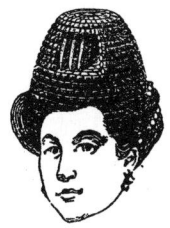

You complain about the chip on my shoulder—I worry about the ax in your hand.

✳

Wisdom isn't newsworthy and the media vampires drink the blood of all hopes.

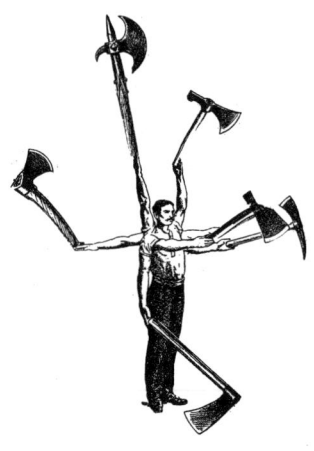

Futility in the morning, despair at noon, devastation at night: next news update 11 p.m.

✳

The essence of happiness: don't give up.

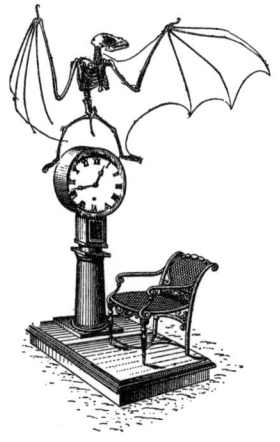

Since insight requires independent thought applied to information, the average American, bloated with the fast food of facts, has grown more informed and more stupid at the same time.

※

What you deem inconvenient may disguise your most formidable adversary.

Better to be exiled in a froZen world than find refuge in a unforgiving mind.

※

Fear stalks the house bereft of love.

As the truth tellers grow more numerous, passionate and articulate, the liars become more organized, cunning and cruel.

✳

Open your mind quickly and your mouth slowly.

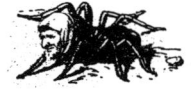

Measure your generosity by your response to selfishness.

※

Perplexity arouses; satisfaction numbs.

Truth cloaks itself in paradox, lies in deception, poetry in obscurity, love in self-effacement. Everything important remains masked.

✳

Those that can no longer be surprised lose the capacity to surprise. By being predictably astonishing, some console themselves.

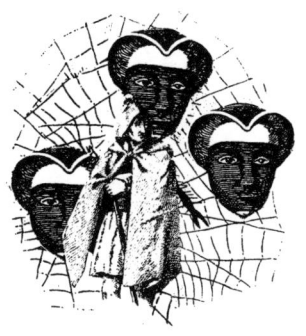

Worries are daydreams without legs, or, worry is the caterpillar, daydream the butterfly.

✳

Joy is the giant, sadness the shadow

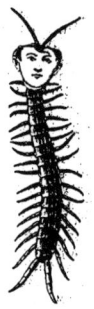

Your shadow's quicksand's will also follow you:
beware the abyss.

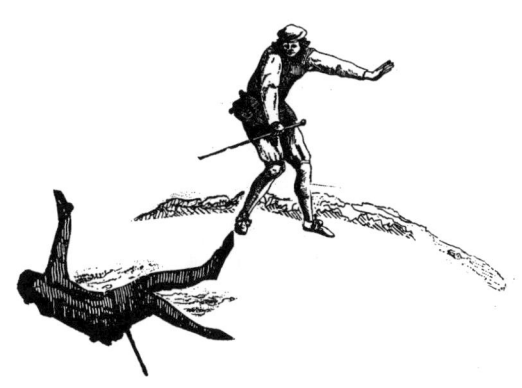

There's more to you than meets the I.

What writing begins only commitment to a point of view completes.

✴

Talk opens a possibility to listening, listening to understanding, understanding to insight, insight to change. But anywhere along the line the chain might break.

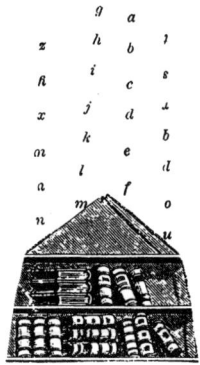

Magic remains invisible and unknown because it must by discovered unconsciously and by accident. It cannot be located, only noticed.

✳

Words descending like snowflakes or rain. A few too many and I think about shelter.

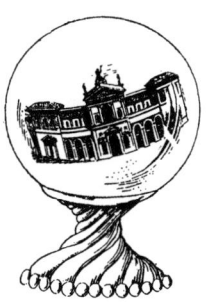

At the heart of some poems there is no meaning but at the heart of every meaning there is a poem.

✳

What hasn't been said in what is said is the part that sings—or stings.

Friends are like angels, wonderfully giving and kind, but mostly invisible or flying off somewhere.

*

If we only knew how much others needed us we might let ourselves need them.

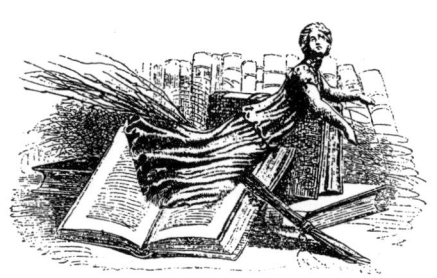

Caring eyes think they can see and do anything. They are right.

＊

Some treasures grow only when they are shared—notably memories.

To treasure—that is the treasure.

*

If you can't find time to do everything find time to do
nothing.

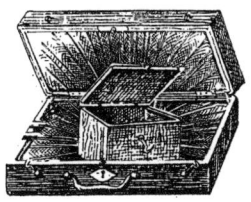

To embrace a truth at the price of one's vanity repays the cost in the coin of equanimity.

＊

Thrive on beginnings, endure endings.

Those who insult themselves all day dislike being slighted, the way an accomplished thief hates being caught.

＊

Just as sorrow covets compassion, vanity craves praise.

A significant error provokes reflection; a major blunder demands change; an impossible dilemma reveals your soul.

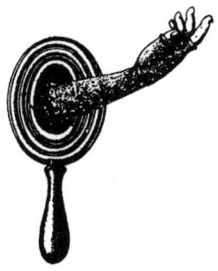

Yesterday was two days before tomorrow.

Nothing is easy until you do it every day.

＊

The secret of generosity is to know how to rest.

When intrusion becomes a right all other rights lack teeth.

✳

I don't care much for birthdays or most holidays. That every day is assigned a number, a first name and a surname, and every moment labeled with another number provides more than enough temporal bureaucracy for me.

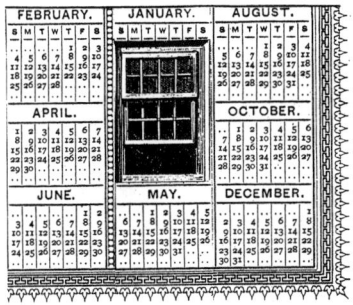

Great success and great compassion are not that compatible: this is why compassionate people find their own failures and that of others worth thinking about.

✳

For contemplatives motivation is like the tides— when they go out, time for a sunbath.

Those that are too easily embarrassed are at the mercy of those that embarrass too easily.

✳

The high tides of triumph recede in the face of the first waves of regret.

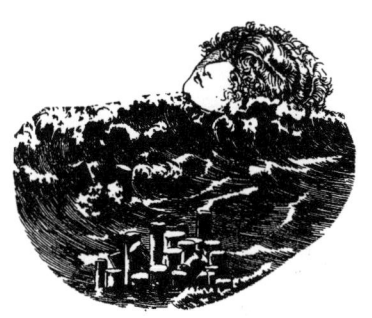

To keep your feet on the ground point your eyes to the sky.

✳

Every good fate includes one long wait.

Through all of our suffering, existence itself shines above it like a star.

✳

What is known to every object and every living thing in the world except human beings is how to be at rest.

There can be no secrets between friends when your silence confides as much as your words.

✻

Coincidence is a wink in the eye of eternity.

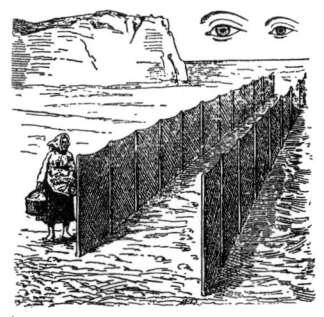

Strength is as important for love as kindness since it is as crucial to challenge the neglect of those whose love we want as it is to challenge our own neglect of those who want our love.

✸

Perhaps before photography, prior to the omnipresence of the pose, people looked—and therefore felt—more like themselves.

Look back—it's always the same. One more moment and you would have found it.

✸

If you haven't asked a question, you haven't said anything.

Empty time is a desert—or an embrace—depending on whether you view it through benign or anxious eyes.

※

We do not dislike ourselves as much as we imagine—we look forward to things knowing one thing for sure—we will be there.

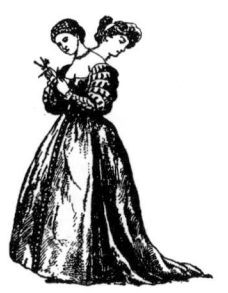

Acknowledge every part and the whole will shine.

✳

To value the useless finds its apotheosis in the farthest realms of art. But this is not the same as feeling useless.

Even what you strongly want to do you must force yourself to do. Why? Because negation is the norm, a creditor waiting to pounce.

✳

Unentangled perseverance produces energy. Energy creates delight. Delight brings happiness. . .

The first inkling is that no one else seems to understand what you want. Then you realize you do not know. Then you know.

✳

The movement of life is like the wind. You can't see it until a breeze comes along and you notice it's there; or it rushes at you suddenly and almost knocks you off your feet.

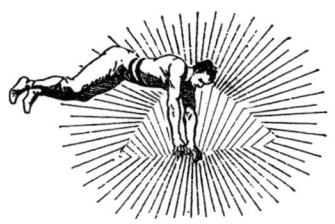

Celebrated names and deeds are so widely remembered, personal help and kindness so readily forgotten.

＊

Earnestness, the child of conscience, is ignored, sarcasm, a descendant of malice, applauded.

If you forget what it is like to go hungry you will forget what it's like to taste anything.

✳

Stumble—discover.

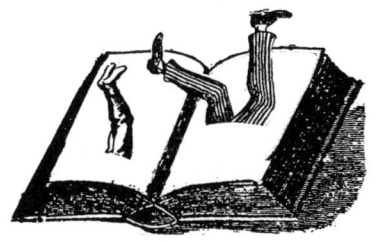

When I see something beautiful I try not to think about poetry; when I see poetry I just try not to think.

※

Never ponder, never sink, never overeat, never drink, never proselytize, never stall, never do anything at all.

There are three things in life well worth waiting for:
sublime passion, a superb meal and an inspired idea.
Right now I'd settle for a good book.

✳

Maturity: the state of mind that allows one to love a
friend even when that friend does not admire one's
writing.

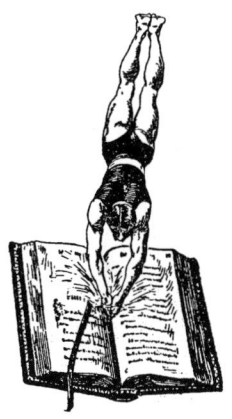

Reading and writing, that begin as thinking's tutor, end as thinking's master.

✳

Take care not to purposely take the wrong step after you have mistakenly blundered into the right one.

The novice plays to the invited guests, the master plays to the gallery.

✳

Listen well to the disputes of the philosophers within yourself, but never sit at their feet.

Your fears encompass as much information about your world as your library.

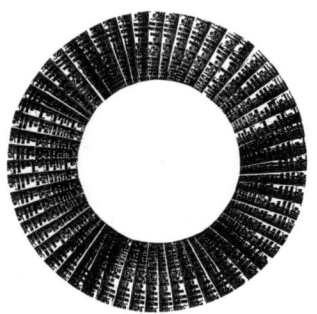

If you make truth a frequent companion, courage will be your friend.

Sometimes the music overwhelms the words,
sometimes the poet overshadows the poem.

*

When one hand envies the other, nothing can be
held.

Our stories are the hands we need to grasp the truths of life and the arms we use to hold it close.

✳

The mind's truth needs fiction's face.

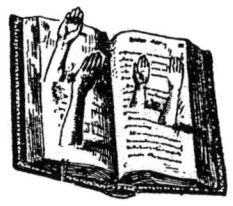

Never reveal what makes you happy, or at least conceal some things, because unless you can be surprised, you will never be loved.

✳

Hidden hearts, like flowers in darkness, wilt quickly.

Self-destruction may feel like rebellion in a society where weakness and doubt are increasingly looked upon as suspect behaviors.

＊

The more contemporary life demands acquiescence and assent, the harder, and more necessary it is to something, anything, solo.

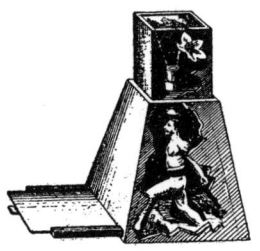

Who can believe the bellowing blasts of bravery's brass band realizing they are mainly meant to crush or subdue the stricken sighs of insignificance within?

※

These days life explodes like a thunderclap but still the clouds move gently.

Nakedness is universally fascinating except for the naked truth—which must be considered boring—since it is always decked out in controversy, or at least wit.

※

Everyone knows what to say—no one knows what to do—except for those who do not care what they say and shoot first.

Mood, reminiscence, hunch, whimsy, expectation, afterthought—silhouettes that flower into portraits.

※

Zero wails like a siren.

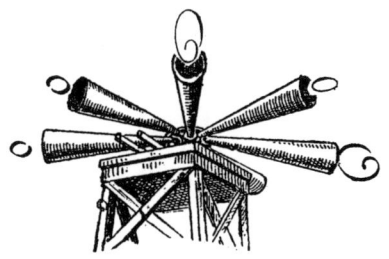

Morning remembers and explains everything but understands and forgives nothing.

＊

Complexity's cautions dance dolefully amidst simplicity's smiling certainties.

Which is more important—the word or the idea? Which is more important—your feet or the ground?

＊

Be decent—dissent.

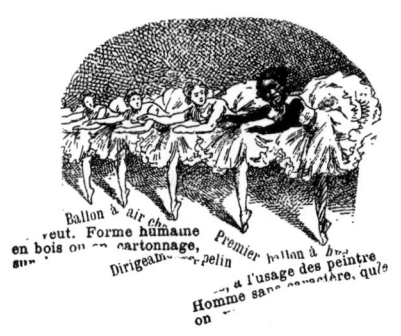

Your doubts might be the seeds of unknown flowers,
if only you would replant them among your ideas
instead of your presentiments.

✳

Words express meanings but their rhythms express
their intentions.

Ask your feet to take you where your mind won't go.

✳

Understanding the world and its needs may tell me
why I should give; but it is understanding myself and
my own needs that tells me why I am able to give.

True, contentment rests within—but it likes to be awakened gently and, even then, only to dance.

*

Admiration visits; love resides.

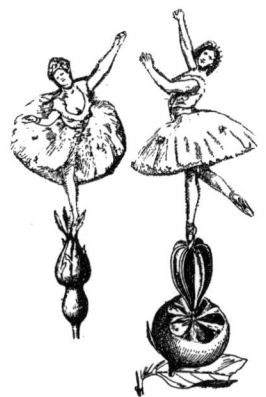

When I am sad I am not myself. A strange being inhabits my body who I don't know and can't recognize.

＊

Worry is hurry with nowhere to go.

The child in us: perpetually impatient, hurried, earnest, astonished.

＊

Nothing ventured, nothing pained.

When I'm outside I feel more inside myself; when I'm inside I look out.

＊

Ahead of myself, behind the others.

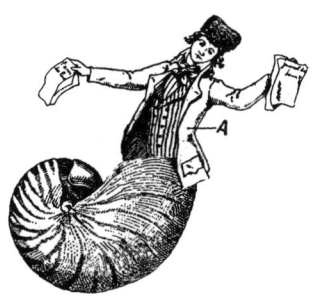

The seductive informalities of contemporary life correspond to the ironic formalisms of contemporary art.

✺

Define me by how I think, describe me by what I know, know me by how I feel.

It is a fine thing to take pleasure in thought but, as with so many other things, we can think too little or too much. Too little produces a mental manikin, too much a chattering puppet.

＊

We never know what we are thinking until we think about it.

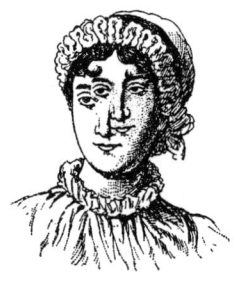

Sadness and joy are not two different songs, but two different refrains of the same song.

✳

When you can't find the time to get lost in thought you lose your mind.

Happiness is a rare guest for those who send infrequent invitations.

✳

The gourmet of happiness is a gourmand of sorrow.

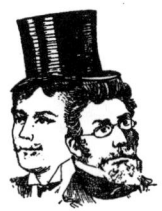

Victors are careful to conceal their disillusionment with the rules of the games they wish to win. "Confidence" is at the heart of this charade.

✳

Artists must get lost in order to discover anything as the freeways lead only to gas stations, malls and parking lots.

Our daily Darwin: in order to sustain itself, happiness must remain oblivious to the unhappiness it creates in others.

＊

Misery commiserates; the American "pursuit of happiness" decimates.

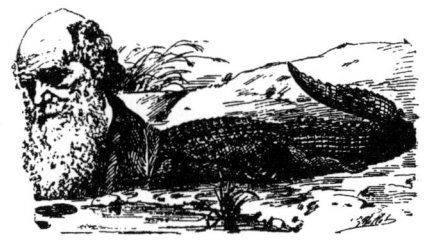

Just as there are shrewd animals who fake death in order to deceive predators, there are artists who feign failure in order to elude imitators. This device does not discourage the bottom feeders, however.

✳

One might as well cloak one's generosity in an air of indifference, since where kindness is viewed as weakness, loneliness prevails.

Up to your neck in shit and sharks, and still thinking of someone's cold and cutting words. . .

✳

In the pharmacopoeia of life, work is the elixir, pleasure the balm.

Anger is a desperate tiger that must be tamed—
befriend or be devoured.

※

The relentless critic hungers for your pride—not your
excellence.

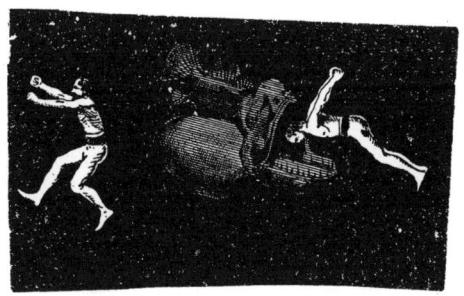

An ounce of insight outweighs a ton of knowledge.

✳

All that titters is not bold.

Listen to the whispers—all the bold voices have had their say.

※

Strategy, shrewdness, brilliance, determination, pride, power, love, all will falter—hope alone remains infallible.

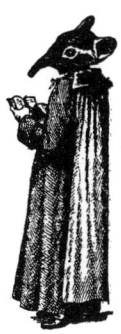

You can always tell how much a well-known writer is being read by how condescending they are. The less read, the more condescending.

＊

No fame without maim.

The unbending competitive drive that facilitates taking pleasure in condescending to or disparaging some, while glorifying others, joins stealing elections, the neo-con crowd, torture and terrorism in that horrific, intractable slide towards dismantling democracy.

＊

Equality plus empathy equals nobility.

Sufficient exaggeration can make any detail of experience fascinating—or frightening—depending on the light.

※

"The best" is the beast.

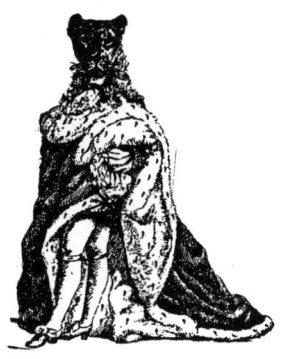

Once again, disappointment performs its ardent solo when suddenly, with a rumble of drums and a burst of violins, the dreamer is released from a melancholy sojourn in the past.

✳

Every feeling evokes its reminiscent melody and its tiny surprise.

The dream of justice is a rare balm for the wounded giant, humankind.

✴

The mean teach the kind how to hide their pain so as to corrupt and enlist them in their ranks.

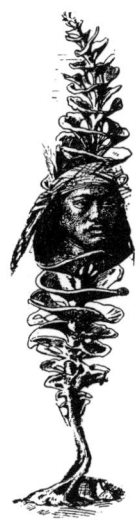

Small disappointments revive the child in us, which would be an equal recompense if we could but see it so.

✳

Those reluctant to disappoint forfeit the talent to surprise.

Delight is the first language to be understood and the last to be forgotten. But from birth until death the meaning of pain rests opaque and obscure whose clearest expression is silence or a scream.

✳

Anyone can think of clever things to say but can you explain to yourself exactly what you were feeling first thing this morning?

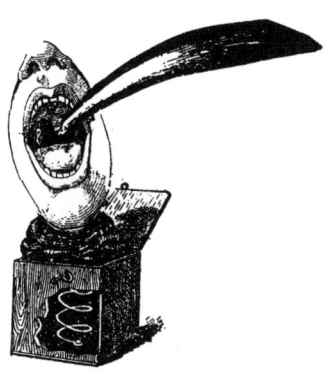

The endless questioning of youth is balanced by the endless answering of age.

✳

Where comparison ends opportunity begins.

A notable difference between being old and being young is that rather than being bored by the calm before storm you enjoy it.

✳

On the whole, people are more tolerant of a criminal than an unhappy person.

As perplexity frequently foreshadows the new,
adoration as often augurs the old.

*

Opinions and affections mixed together, like vinegar
and oil, may spice something bland, but left to
themselves they quickly separate.

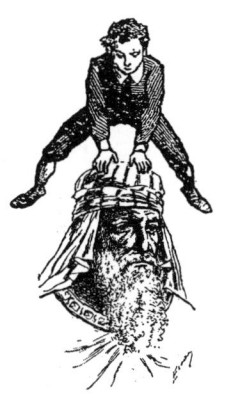

The only things worth being understood in what we say are those things we make clear in what others have said.

✹

Truths about poetry are the keys that unlock the cages. You are there to watch the birds fly away and when they go you never think twice about the truth, the keys or the cages.

Those who do not listen are usually the most desperate to be heard and the least concerned about whether they were.

✹

Thought is what remains after all the interruptions.

Life's conspiracy—perhaps the shadow of desire—an irrepressible aura of incompletion.

✳

What you are thinking is the parrot in the cage of what you are doing.

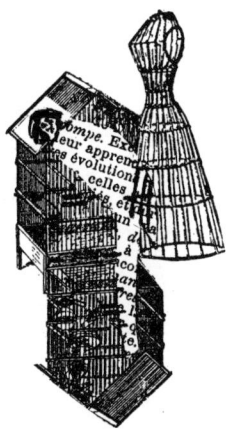

Draw contentment from mundane repetition, find a refuge from strident surprise.

※

Too much satisfaction in approbation, too much affliction in disparagement or indifference.

Imitating well is the sincerest form of revenge.

※

Slow and steady comes in like a lamb and gets fleeced by a lion.

There is no firm feeling of accomplishment until your friend has emphatically explained to you all the reasons you should have it.

✳

It is one thing to appropriate some ideas here and there, but it is completely another to lack the means to discover your own.

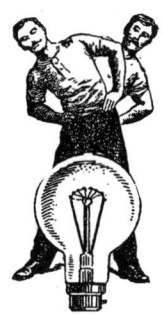

News and advertising persuade us to memorize what we can't believe.

＊

Truth is bland, so few ask for seconds; surprise is sweet and everyone asks for more.

The admirable attributes of who and what you love have captured your devotion but it is the enigmatic qualities you think about.

＊

Originality is impossible where imitation is universal.

The jagged peaks of judgment provide a provisional
bastion beyond a condescending chorus of criticism.

✳

Opinion rarely sings solo.

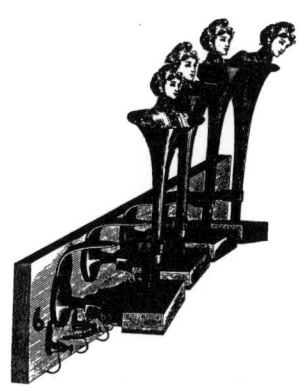

For very long I have been alienated by the expectable. Now I am additionally alienated by the expectable alienation by the expectable.

※

What did all that running ahead of myself accomplish other than declaiming emphatically: "Nothing can stop me!"

In a world parched by desiccated words and empty lies, silence sounds sweet.

※

Those who always know where they are going are not very interesting when they get there.

It's comfort—not conscience—that makes cowards of us all.

＊

The bland leading the bland. . .

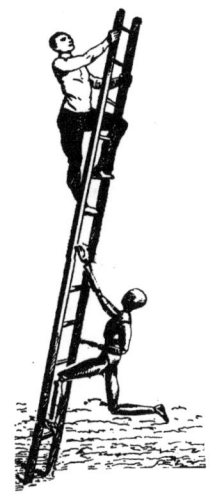

Wit is used more often to silence than to say.

※

Something will happen—meanwhile, just live.

In the voice of kindness truth sings, or at least rings; from the mouth of cruelty it stings.

※

Children can keep hardly anything to themselves. It's love that should be seen and not heard.

Malice is spoken in countless barbed dialects and a single lenient one: silence.

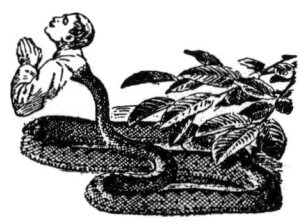

Open ridicule wounds; silent derision poisons.

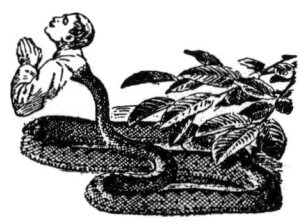

As a child they looked up to them, and later straight in the eye; in their middle years smiled smugly down on them; now they shake their heads and sigh.

＊

Modesty protects friendship, pride destroys it.

It is intelligent to despise stupidity yet even more intelligent to comprehend it.

＊

The weak respect cunning more than kindness yet the cunning know they are more feared than loved. So—in time—the cunning get weak from loneliness while the kind grow strong with trust.

The smile of an ambitious soul rarely assures a safe haven.

✳

Frequent disappointment, deception and betrayal induce the kind and warm to join the ranks of the cold and cautious.

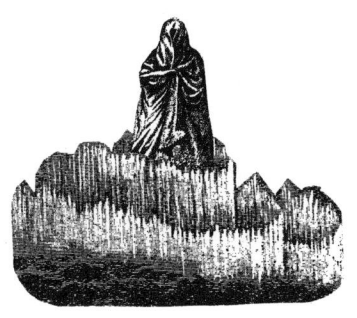

Beware the sly generosity of the thief who freely distributes the right to steal.

✸

If someone takes what is yours you have less, but if you forfeit your generosity you lose everything.

Those compelled to mock the serious are perhaps not quite sure who will get the last laugh.

✸

You thought you were completely free of scorn until someone's shaft of ridicule pierced your poise.

Flattery and deceit paint a fine smile on imitation's lips in deception's hall of mirrors.

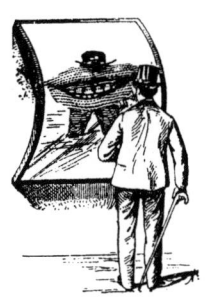

The lighthouse is far away and dim on the shores of mistrust's lonely latitudes.

Powerful feelings perpetuate themselves by means of a trick—they promise—or threaten—to expand infinitely and eternally. Through moods, they try to install themselves indefinitely. But a mood is a replica of an emotion, only a product of the feelings that generated it.

✳

An hour of regret is enough for three lifetimes.

Even when today's novels, stories and poems eliminate the plots they never eradicate the twists.

✳

I think I found what I was looking for: looking for.

Traditions harden into conventions when memory and empathy are replaced by reverence and the cold devotion that supports it.

✳

There can be a useful tradition of unconventionality but conventional unconventionality is a travesty that subverts its entire aim.

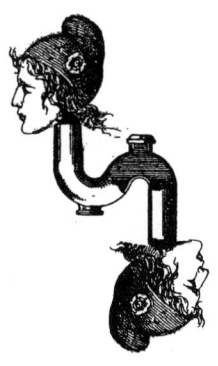

Sun, water and praise will grow anything.

✳

The only thing in this world that is infinite is the envy of small minds.

There is one mountain that will never be scaled: the height of arrogant stupidity.

✳

When you've been duped do something quickly, but make your plan slowly.

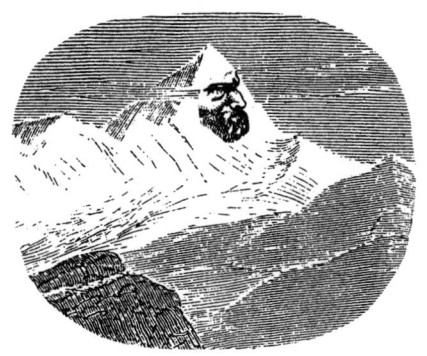

When cooking up ideas let ambition be the flame and patience the chef.

＊

Gratitude is the child of kindness and the blossom of wisdom.

Truth might visit the solitary but you will rarely find liars alone.

＊

Life is the desert, truth the oasis.

Fame is a restless, fickle friend whose flame is greatest near its end.

*

Those fruits of thought that ripen slowly are eaten quickly.

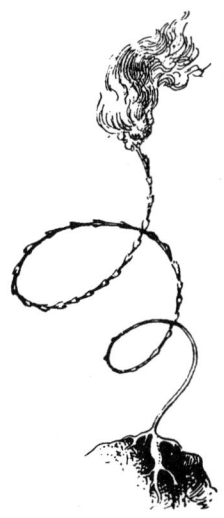

The fewer the notes the greater the melody.

✳

Originality—having the boldness to exhale what everyone else inhales.

Remember music, particularly in times of weariness and despair—as its charms are nearly inexhaustible and its demands negligible.

✳

Aimless thought explores every open path—but most converge on the downward slope.

Like so many other endeavors in contemporary life, music too often tries to subdue the beasts instead of charming them like Debussy.

✳

A light touch may not hold things as long—yet this way they are more likely to return.

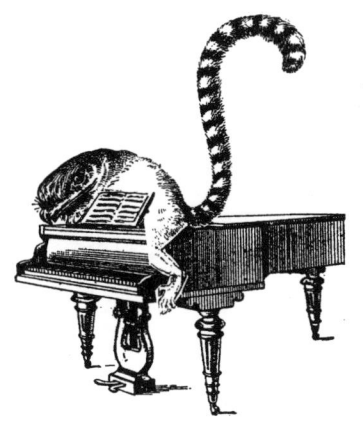

Everything is going downhill so fast—but we'll need the momentum—the next slope could be the steepest one yet.

＊

God created the world in 7 days—3 of them waiting to get online, 2 to clear out the spam, 1 to download and 1 to rest.

The deeper you dig the harder the rock, the narrower the tunnel, the lonelier the journey.

✺

Steadiness of purpose and enjoyment of life form an odd, yet incomparable, friendship.

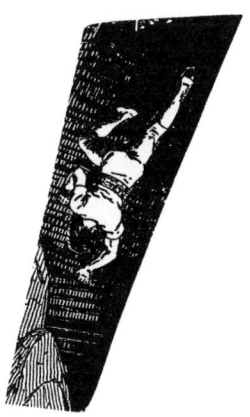

Until you try hope remains in limited supply.

＊

Let your arms grow longer every day and there will be more to hold.

In the heart of your wound, find your path.

＊

Suffering shouts, happiness whispers.

The more you know what's new the less you learn what's true.

✳

To know is more enlightening, but less comforting, than to be known.

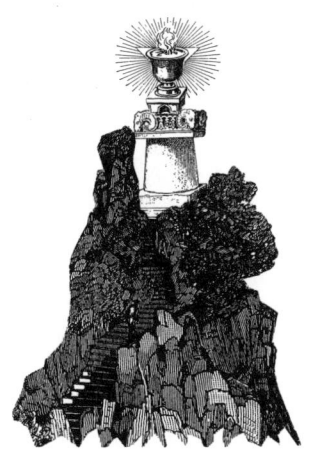

Worry wonders; courage laughs.

✳

Knowledge leads to wisdom but courage finds it.

The recognition of something's value frequently leads to little more than creating more desire for it. This is how an appetite for acquisition trumps the progression of discernment.

✳

Knowledge without insight is like humor without wit.

The long journey shorter, the heavy load lighter, temper tamed—forget yourself.

✳

That fool is wise who forgot everything except how to laugh.

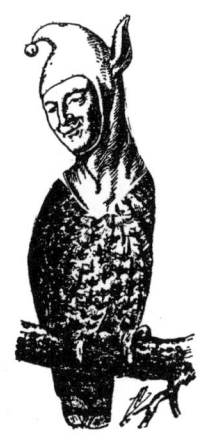

Without daydreams between them, experiences themselves tend to become overly dreamlike—one displacing another suddenly and with too much logic—like sequences in a film, inexorable and coming to the point too soon.

※

Ideas come together the way a body makes itself comfortable. Somewhere, perhaps in the throat, a shoulder or an arm the thought resides. The thought is a link between fragments that might fit together— that want to be together—so they remain immobile until they unite and escape by means of the voice.

When a "raison d'etre" fades it is hard to recall why
we did what we did. Remembering appears linked to
what made something "apropos".

✳

Think or, better yet, daydream around, among,
between—in the interstices—and not a moment will
be wasted.

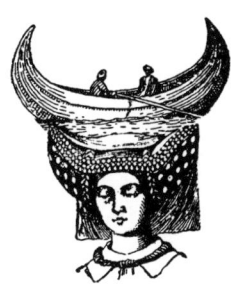

One by one the finest philosophers concluded
they should no longer try to tell us how to live.
Imperceptibly, yet gradually, an immense sadness fell
upon the world and the sadists took over.

❋

Think for yourself or go mad with everyone.

Effervescent writing, like its cousins beer and champagne, should be consumed all at once or fast as its bubbles also quickly disappear.

✳

Enthusiasm's effort builds a castle out of hopes; with a careless elbow, antagonism levels the playing field.

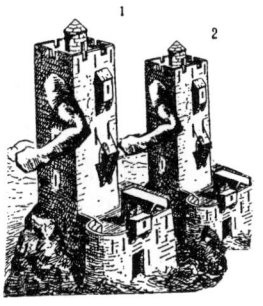

Take care not to acquire too many cold friends, as you must become like them. In this realm cold transfers more quickly than warmth, and more permanently.

✳

In people coldness has the advantage of anaesthetizing pain. These folks take the greatest delight in their ambitions and their advantages over others, despite whatever generosity they put on display.

Feelings are not the threat, or shouldn't be. To the extent that I feel gratitude and affection, I should also expect to feel outrage and antipathy. Indifference is the true threat, the outcome of deadening.

✳

Someone responds, I respond. If you ignore me, how can I fail, eventually, to ignore you? Nevertheless, each of us is aware the other is out there, somewhere.

The sun shines equally on lovers and the heartless.

✳

On a moonless night, my fears, disguised as friends, whisper threats.

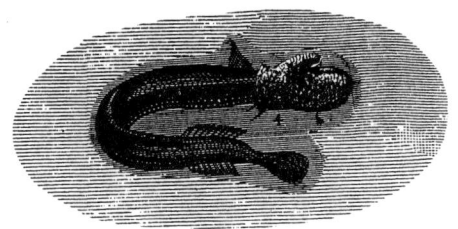

Tell your troubles to a dark cloud you get rain.

＊

Cold latitudes proffer cold platitudes.

The wise philosophize well but are lax about
the obvious; dolts are inarticulate but wary and
watchful. Who rules?

＊

The warmer the luck the colder the attitude.

Again you were challenged by that callous friend—
who always inquires how you are when you meet—
but never seems to notice how you feel when you
part.

✳

Solve global cooling global warming will follow.

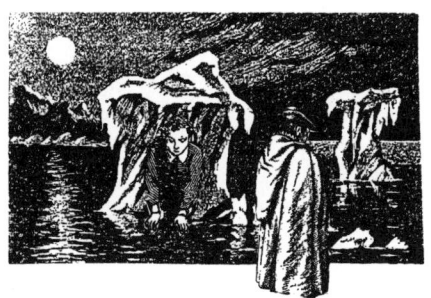

The truth can take a bite out of life, but it cannot taste it.

✳

Like the weather, the truth can harm—which is why you need shelter.

To wish to do the things you have to do creates energy and invites contentment.

✳

Sharpen your mind's teeth on your mistakes.

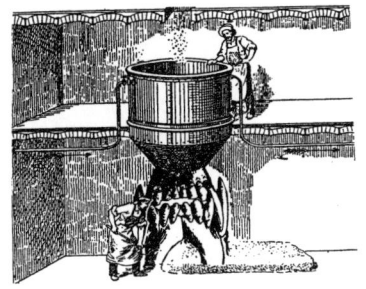

The truth that affirms is quoted; the truth that surprises is discussed, the truth that wounds is remembered; the truth that helps is understood.

✳

What is done for its own sake survives the drought and then the storm.

The complacent regard the truth the way some regard a panorama of sky: too obvious for these, too distant for those.

✳

Even the useless isn't useless.

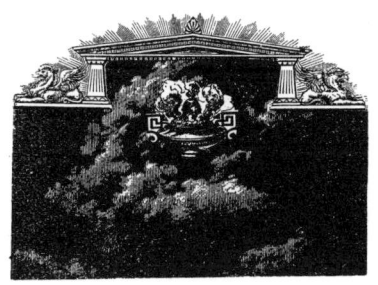

What is the difference between being very patient about the suffering of someone you care about and being indifferent to it? Shouldn't we insist on the other's attempt at happiness—or at least try and make them laugh?

※

Because it is so ubiquitous and yet so transformative, persistence in caring remains largely invisible. The results are sometimes noticed but these are usually ascribed to something special about the recipient.

Rise above the petty thoughts which viewed as pains
will unite into chains.

＊

Anger, hurt and cruelty, helpless without each other,
will soon subside.

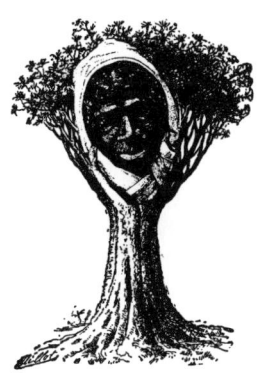

Love restores hope, hope imagination, imagination memory, memory emotion, emotion song.

*

Truth is a ladder composed of painful steps but at the top one you see from the sky.

As writers climb the ladder to success they are wise to shed their feelings, since the clouds, that appear so substantial from below, from above appear flat and lonely because there is room for only one. This is a dilemma for their readers, who expect to feel things in order to be convinced the work remains substantial.

＊

Friendship is a game of chess that should be played more gently and appreciatively as time goes on, otherwise the opponents will deprive themselves of the partners who have so steadily inspired them.

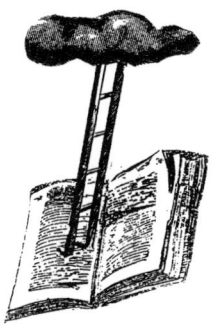

Greed is the opium of the swindler; indifference is the armor of the weary and oppressed.

✳

No sky, no smile; no smile, no sky.

When others do not want what you have to give, should this stop you from getting what you want to give?

✳

When life is confusing for those who think for themselves, the confused are running the show.

About the same time a generation of men perceive
how uncertain their fathers are they prepare for war.

✳

Violence enrages but the numb and frozen aftermath
is silent.

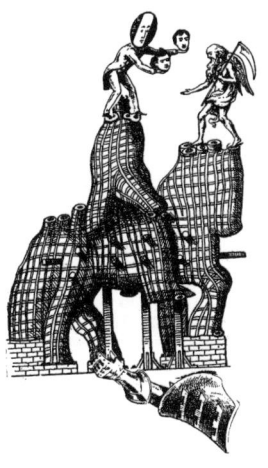

Tried and true convictions don't raise heads but they don't lower minds either.

＊

Convictions without empathy can justify anything.

Principle and perfection have facilitated more pain and harm than anger and failure will ever imagine.

✺

The devil's in the details—the beauty too.

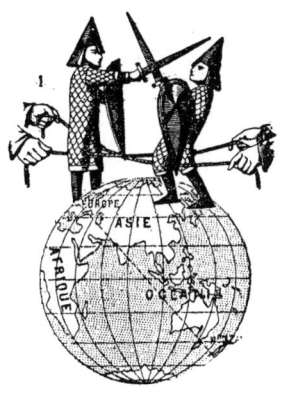

To tolerate one's own suffering or that of others without trying or at least wishing to reduce it is itself a kind of evil because, as suffering grows, so does evil.

✳

Celebrities who are prolific and talk freely inspire affection because they give the impression that at any moment they might blurt out the secrets of their success.

What has eroded with time is not so much the pleasure of discovering the truth but awareness of the pleasure in confronting its nemesis.

✳

Not only is truth stranger than fiction but it is stranger than facts.

Human intelligence contains a flaw that waters the seeds of its own destruction: impatience.

※

Artists and intellectuals bribe patrons and politicians with mirages of progress.

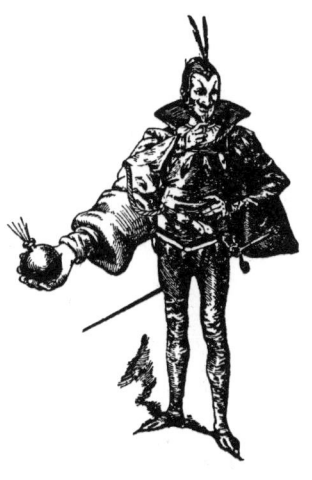

If the essence of life consists of learning to love, why wouldn't every other effort to offer lasting pleasure be guided by the same principle?

✳

Unless accompanied by an ability to love, thinking is mostly painful.

Curiosity battles with boredom but love defeats it.

✳

Even the heaviest burdens are buoyant on love's wings.

The wisest of all are wise in love and they are fools.

✳

Memories are silhouettes of love or the shadows of
its absence.

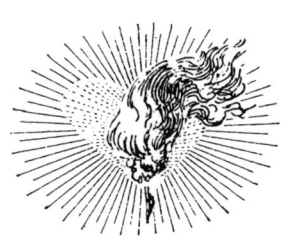

An exceptional appreciation of the ordinary is the source of much that is extraordinary.

❋

Those sophists who dismiss every illusion are also blind to every miracle.

The interminable night of rage shuns the mirror in the morning.

❋

Hatred seeks contempt but escapes kindness.

Kindness might be blindness when the cruel rule.

✳

Good brings about evil by angering the cruel; evil creates good by alarming the kind.

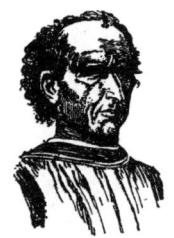

Everything is pushing my buttons today—except the one that says "on."

✳

Peace and quiet—there goes the diet.

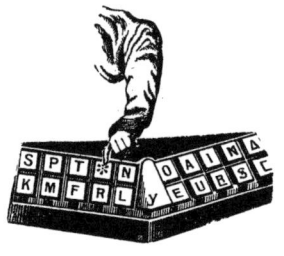

Even more ghastly than hatred itself, indifferent eyes fly by coldly like headlights of cars on dark streets at night.

＊

Convictions contingent on praise fade with the earliest qualms.

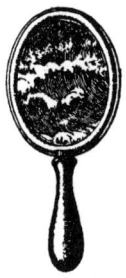

Even when being hurtful, people think they've been kind. They could have been so much meaner!

※

The best way to show how you feel is to ask a question.

Regarding mistakes with a degree of tolerant affection lessens worry and enhances change.

※

Spend your whole life annoyed with the rules of others or take a few moments creating your own.

The ever vigilant ape within us (who remains, only out of sheer compassion) continues to protect us, in spite of ourselves; knowing full well that—out of vanity—we will deny its very existence should it reveal its face to us, or anyone else, even for an instant.

✳

Our affection for the books we love is similar to that of a parent for a child—as much for the fact that they are likely to outlive us as for the qualities we hold so dear.

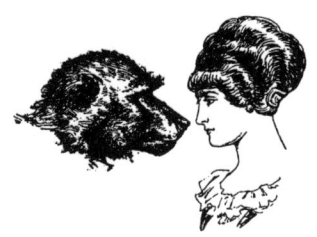

Writers and thieves have something in common—to succeed they must dispose of the evidence.

✳

You don't go to masters for correct techniques but for efficacious attitudes.

After you've read poetry long enough, with each successive reading you understand more of the magician's tricks. At this stage you read more to understand the poet than the poem because poets have infinitely more tricks up their sleeves than their poems.

✳

Confess you were wrong and gain affection—profess you were right and lose it.

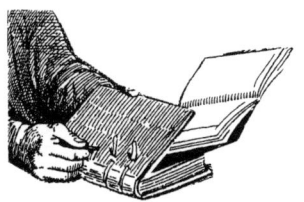

The perpetual satisfaction taken in accomplishments stems from believing they are among your rival's greatest torments; yet soon you begin suspecting they might be one of the competition's greatest spurs.

※

Where pride fails doubt prevails.

Envy would not be such a bad thing, except that we always envy the wrong one.

※

To know how to begin things, and mostly see them through, yet still enjoy the suspense between, is a secret shared by few.

Decision's pendulum can seem slow—but let it sway until you know.

*

Cynical, wary—alert, prepared; vulnerable, earnest—dreamy, astonished.

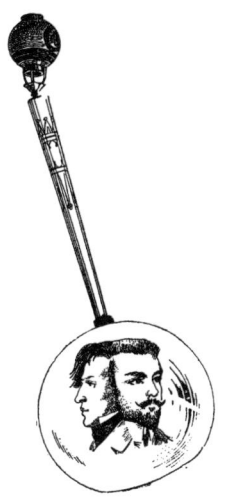

If you are a male, the preponderance of other males will find a way to condescend to you, even with their dying breath. A panhandler will tell you to "have a nice day"—as if it were theirs to give—or accept your donation with the indifference of a king.

*

Intelligent response is to acclamation as love is to sex. As the latter grows ever more prevalent and public, the former grows ever more private and rare.

Treating others as equals demands considerable stamina. Most people prefer to worship and be worshipped—thus the predictable failure of democracies.

✳

No one would credit anyone for anything if not for the compulsive craving for hierarchy.

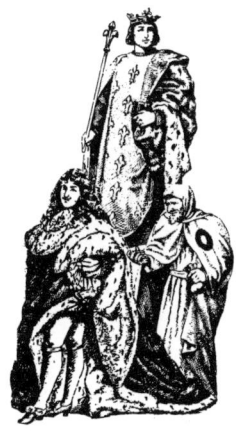

People drive each other crazy more or less continuously and then deliberate and debate about how others should behave.

＊

You could multiply the dictionary by a thousand and still not have enough words to describe what most people think and feel in a single day.

I read to understand feelings.
I write to understand thoughts.
Sometimes talking helps me to understand what I need to know or do. But if I want to just understand I stay quiet.

＊

Understanding is like gladly coming to the end of a chapter of a book you've been totally absorbed in. But still, you don't want the book to end.

As you reach that moment in life when time becomes more crucial than anything, you are induced to invoke philosophy, if only by default.

＊

Seduced by hope or conquered by despair, animated by energy or cloaked in flair.

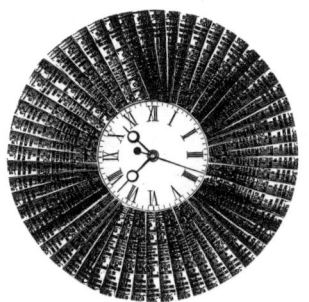

I never stop learning because I never stop making mistakes, or having to deal with the mistakes of others.

＊

The old love the morning when life begins again; the young love the night they think will never end.

Sadness offers a hundred words and explanations while happiness has but few and is inexplicable.

＊

It is easier to lose love than passion, but it is sadder to lose passion.

Anyone can easily appear supremely sophisticated and all-knowing by understating or withholding their reactions. Like death, another masterful leveler, silence obliterates all distinction by remaining cool and unimpressed.

※

Irony, the shield and sword of literary politics, ends its days living alone on one side of the moon, while its polar opposite, sentimentality, assumes its solo residence on the other.

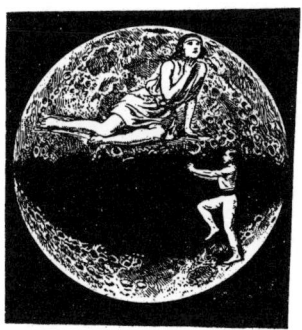

Two steps forward, one step horizontal.

✳

The perennial paradox: impatient to finish it, wishing it wouldn't end.

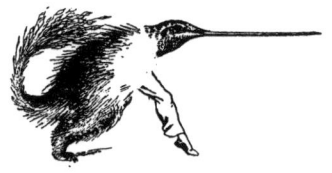

It is good to possess at least a nominal acceptance of reality. It doesn't make life easier, or longer, but it does make it funnier.

✴

To know what interests oneself is half of success; to know what interests others is all of it.

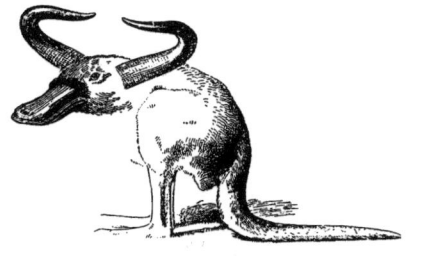

The center will not hold—no matter —everything is
in orbit anyway—keep turning.

✳

Celebrate your sensitivity—don't be numb. The
greatest danger in the world's ever increasing
intrusiveness lies in accepting it.

Every moment you have ever lived lives on, and will one day visit or receive you, if only you would make it welcome.

※

Ride Pegasus hard into the present so its wings can sweep the future and the past.

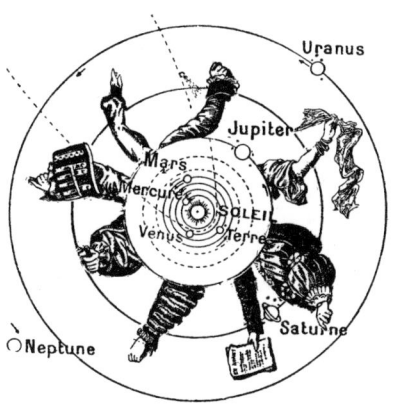

Our glimpse of life is from a train going fast: where we can barely distinguish the present from the past.

✳

Love is watered by truth at its roots but its arms reach up towards light and kindness.

There's no time for remembering—savor everything
to the quick.

❋

Everything gets clearer and clearer—then you realize
you don't have to understand.

If you speak in a voice too low no one will hear you. If you speak in one too loud no one will listen. If you say too little no one will understand. If you say too much, no one will care to understand.

✳

As with everything else of significance, happiness must be pieced together gradually, like a jig-saw puzzle—only to be pulled apart and put together again and again.

To acknowledge your feelings is to sometimes feel unsure. To ignore your feelings is to always feel unsure.

✳

To those who can listen, even the melody of sadness lingers.

The pleasure in viewing the belongings of the great masters derives from the inability to believe that they did things in the same way and places that everyone else does.

※

My father never spoke so now I won't stop listening.

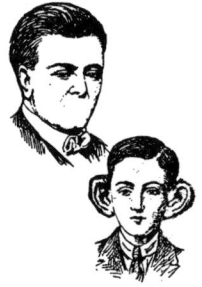

The poems are all telling me the same thing. "This is all a poem. You're alive, get it?"

＊

Ah, poetry. It's such a pleasure to have something that does not demand to be understood, in a world where clearly there is already not one iota of understanding to spare.

As you read further into the past writers were more often hopeful yet desperately earnest; as you come closer to the present they are more often hopeless but desperately funny.

✳

To span the space between the known and the unknown begin with the gulf between the thought and the said.

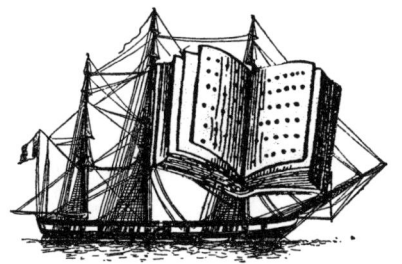

Much of our experience of others and their experience remains foreign to us. We must internally translate or we are doomed to misunderstand or be misunderstood.

✳

Listening better is frequently the best answer one can give.

Everyone behaves like an idiot from time to time but only the honest ones ever think about it.

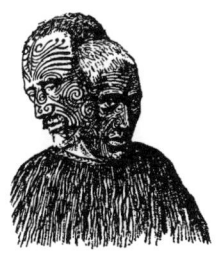

If compassion won acclaim life would be art.

People go to extremes in order to be different. But the remarkable differences are the subtle ones.

✳

Life creates immense variety—but all endings are the same.

No two thoughts are exactly alike—until someone writes them down.

✳

All books exist to end in a thought.

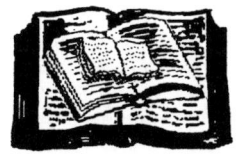

THE AMERICA AWARDS
for a lifetime contribution to international writing
Awarded by the Contemporary Arts Educational Project, Inc.
in loving memory of Anna Fahrni

The 2009 Award winner is:

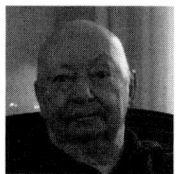

GÜNTER KUNERT (GDR/GERMANY) 1929

PREVIOUS WINNERS:
1994 Aimé Cesaire [Martinique] 1913–2008
1995   Harold Pinter [England] 1930–2008
1996 José Donoso [Chile] 1924-1996 (awarded prior to his death)
1997 Friederike Mayröcker [Austria] 1924
1998 Rafael Alberti [Spain] 1902-1999
1999 Jacques Roubaud [France] 1932
2000 Eudora Welty [USA] 1909-2001
2001 Inger Christensen [Denmark] 1935–2009
2002 Peter Handke [Austria] 1942
2003 Adonis (Ali Ahmad Said) [Syria/Lebanon] 1930
2004 José Saramago [Portugal] 1922
2005 Andrea Zanzotto [Italy] 1921
2006 Julien Gracq (Louis Poirier) [France] 1910-2007
2007 Paavo Haavikko [Finland] 1931
2008 John Ashbery [USA] 1927

The rotating panel for The America Awards currently consists of Douglas Messerli [chairman], Will Alexander, Luigi Ballerini, Charles Bernstein, Peter Constantine, Peter Glassgold, Deborah Meadows, Martin Nakell, John O'Brien, Marjorie Perloff, Dennis Phillips, Joe Ross, Jerome Rothenberg, Paul Vangelisti, and Mac Wellman